THE POCKET VITAMIN GUIDE

SUSAN KAGEN PODELL
M.S., R.D.

MAIN STREET BOOKS
DOUBLEDAY
New York London Toronto
Sydney Auckland

A MAIN STREET BOOK
PUBLISHED BY DOUBLEDAY
a division of Bantam Doubleday Dell Publishing Group, Inc.
1540 Broadway, New York, New York 10036

MAIN STREET BOOKS, DOUBLEDAY, and the portrayal of a building with a tree are trademarks of Doubleday, a division of Bantam Doubleday Dell Publishing Group, Inc.

Library of Congress Cataloging-in-Publication Data
Podell, Susan Kagen.
The pocket vitamin guide / Susan Kagen Podell.—
1st ed.
p. cm.
1. Vitamins in human nutrition—Handbooks, manuals, etc.
I. Title.
QP771.P6 1994
612.3′99—dc20 93-2344
CIP

ISBN 0-385-46823-7

Printed in the United States of America
February 1994
FIRST EDITION

Contents

Read any magazine or newspaper, watch TV, or listen to the radio . . . there is advice everywhere about foods we should *avoid* eating to help reduce the risk of disease. But what about what we should eat? Good health is affected by what we include in our diets as well as by what we limit. This is where VITAMINS come in. Vitamins positively affect our health, vitality, and well-being. In fact, we can't live without them!

What Are Vitamins?

Vitamins are organic substances, essential in tiny amounts to regulate every body function. We need them to grow, reproduce, and maintain good health. They are transient helpers that are either used up or stored away for later use. They tend to work in teams doing everything from depositing calcium in bones and aiding in muscle contraction and nerve conduction, to making red blood cells and helping clot blood.

So far, thirteen vitamins have been identified. Four of these are called fat soluble (vitamins A, D, E, and K) because they are found and stored in the fatty parts of food and body tissue. The other nine are called water soluble—vitamin C, thiamin (B_1), riboflavin (B_2), niacin (B_3), vitamin B_6, pantothenic acid, folic acid, biotin, and vitamin B_{12}—and are not stored for any significant time in any body tissue. Water-soluble vitamins that are in excess of the body's needs are generally excreted in the urine. Small amounts, however, are stored for a short time.

Vitamins seem to do everything. But closer observation reveals that their most important functions can be divided into three categories: (1) building the body, (2) protecting the body, and (3) regulating energy production.

Vitamins A, B_6, B_{12}, C, D, and folic acid work to build the body—help make new cells, strong bones, and maintain skin and collagen. Another important function of vitamins A and C, as well as vitamin E, is protecting the body via the immune system and keeping skin and other tissues healthy. Vitamin K has a special protective function in helping clot blood. The most important function of the B vitamins (thiamin, riboflavin, niacin, pantothenic acid, and biotin) is turning food into energy, or energy regulation.

Even though we can't live without them, our bodies cannot make most vitamins. Exceptions include vitamin D, which is manufactured in the skin during exposure to sunlight, and vitamin K, biotin, and pantothenic acid, which are made in the intestines by the normal bacteria that live there. So most vitamins must be supplied in your daily diet. We *don't* need large quantities, however. In all, our daily vitamin requirement amounts to about an eighth of a teaspoon!

♦

Recommended Dietary Allowances: How Much Do We Need?

The general allowance guidelines for vitamins are called the Recommended Dietary Allowance, or RDA. A group of experts based in Washington, D.C., at the National Academy of Science—National Research Council has determined how much of each vitamin people require. The following table shows the RDA for each vitamin.

Do not confuse the RDAs with nutritional requirements. RDAs are only estimates that always *exceed* the vitamin requirements of most healthy people, and they do not apply to every case. For example, people who have special nutritional needs as a result of disease, medication use, or poor health habits will require more.

FOOD AND NUTRITION BOARD, NATIONAL ACADEMY OF SCIENCES—NATIONAL RESEARCH COUNCIL RECOMMENDED DIETARY ALLOWANCES,[a] Revised 1989

Designed for the maintenance of good nutrition of practically all healthy people in the United States

		Fat-Soluble Vitamins				Water-Soluble Vitamins						
Category	Age (years) or Condition	A (μg RE)[b]	D (μg)[c]	E (mg α-TE)[d]	K (μg)	C (mg)	Thiamin (mg)	Riboflavin (mg)	Niacin (mg NE)[e]	B_6 (mg)	Folate (μg)	B_{12} (μg)
Infants	0.0–0.5	375	7.5	3	5	30	0.3	0.4	5	0.3	25	0.3
	0.5–1.0	375	10	4	10	35	0.4	0.5	6	0.6	35	0.5
Children	1–3	400	10	6	15	40	0.7	0.8	9	1.0	50	0.7
	4–6	500	10	7	20	45	0.9	1.1	12	1.1	75	1.0
	7–10	700	10	7	30	45	1.0	1.2	13	1.4	100	1.4
Males	11–14	1,000	10	10	45	50	1.3	1.5	17	1.7	150	2.0
	15–18	1,000	10	10	65	60	1.5	1.8	20	2.0	200	2.0
	19–24	1,000	10	10	70	60	1.5	1.7	19	2.0	200	2.0
	25–50	1,000	5	10	80	60	1.5	1.7	19	2.0	200	2.0
	51+	1,000	5	10	80	60	1.2	1.4	15	2.0	200	2.0

Females	11–14	800	10	8	45	50	1.1	1.3	15	1.4	150	2.0
	15–18	800	10	8	55	60	1.1	1.3	15	1.5	180	2.0
	19–24	800	10	8	60	60	1.1	1.3	15	1.6	180	2.0
	25–50	800	5	8	65	60	1.1	1.3	15	1.6	180	2.0
	51+	800	5	8	65	60	1.0	1.2	13	1.6	180	2.0
Pregnant		800	10	10	65	70	1.5	1.6	17	2.2	400	2.2
Lactating	1st 6 months	1,300	10	12	65	95	1.6	1.8	20	2.1	280	2.6
	2nd 6 months	1,200	10	11	65	90	1.6	1.7	20	2.1	260	2.6

Source: Food and Nutrition Board, National Academy of Sciences—National Research Council, 1989.

[a] The allowances, expressed as average daily intakes over time, are intended to provide for individual variations among most normal persons as they live in the United States under usual environmental stresses. Diets should be based on a variety of common foods in order to provide other nutrients for which human requirements have been less well defined.

[b] Retinol equivalents. 1 retinol equivalent = 1 μg retinol or 6 μg β-carotene.

[c] As cholecalciferol. 10 μg cholecalciferol = 400 IU of vitamin D.

[d] α -Tocopherol equivalents. 1 mg d-α tocopherol = 1 α-TE.

[e] 1 NE (niacin equivalent) is equal to 1 mg of niacin or 60 mg of dietary tryptophan.

The most common vitamins that Americans lack in their daily diet are vitamins A, C, and, in women, B_6. Vitamins A and C are in short supply because most Americans don't eat enough fruits and vegetables, the main sources of these vitamins. For women, vitamin B_6 requirements are fairly high, and thus it is difficult for most women to eat enough to reach their needs. For more information on vitamins A, B_6, and C, see pages 27–33.

◆

Food for Full Vitamin Power

To translate the RDAs into real food and to build a nutritious, vitamin-complete diet, select food from the following groups, in the amount specified.

MEAT AND PROTEIN FOODS

KEY VITAMINS: thiamin, niacin, vitamins B_6 and B_{12}, and pantothenic acid (necessary to turn food into energy and help build body tissue).

One serving is 3 ounces or about the size of the palm of your hand or a deck of cards, or the size of the portion described. Eat two servings every day. Limit high-fat and processed meats such as hot dogs, bologna, sausage, ribs, chicken wings, and bacon.

Lean beef, lamb, pork, and veal
Skinless poultry
Seafood including any fish or shellfish
Eggs—up to four per week (high in cholesterol)
1 cup canned baked beans
1 cup cooked dried beans and peas
1 cup tofu
3 Tbsp peanut butter (high in fat)

MILK AND MILK PRODUCTS

KEY VITAMINS: Vitamins A, B_{12}, D, riboflavin, biotin, and pantothenic acid (necessary to build and protect the body as well as turn food into energy).

One serving is the size of the portion described. Have three or four servings every day. If you can't digest the sugar in milk or are lactose intolerant, you can buy special products in the dairy section. Limit high-fat dairy products and nondairy milk substitutes.

1 cup milk: lowfat, skim, powdered, or buttermilk
1 cup yogurt

1 cup lowfat cottage cheese
Two 1-inch cubes cheese
1 cup pudding or custard
1½ cups soup made with lowfat milk
1 cup ice milk or lowfat ice cream

FRUITS AND VEGETABLES

KEY VITAMINS: Vitamins A, B_6, C, folic acid, and biotin (necessary to protect and build body tissue).

One serving is the size of the portion described. Eat AT LEAST five servings daily.

Fresh or frozen vegetables are best; fresh, frozen, or canned fruits are okay too. Avoid fried vegetables such as french fries or tempura. Limit fruit drinks with added sugar; real fruit juice has more of the vitamins you need.

Vitamin-A Rich Fruits and Vegetables

1 cup spinach, collard greens, kale, mustard greens, or bok choy
2 small apricots
¼ cantaloupe
½ cup carrots, raw or cooked
1 mango
½ cup winter squash
1 sweet potato or yam
1 medium tomato

Vitamin-C Rich Fruits and Vegetables

1 orange
½ grapefruit
½ cup orange or grapefruit juice
¾ cup strawberries
1 papaya
1 kiwifruit
1 cup brussels sprouts
1 cup broccoli
1 cup cauliflower
½ cup green pepper

Others

1¼ cups watermelon
1 small banana
1 apple
2 Tbsp dried fruit
½ cup eggplant
½ cup green beans
½ cup green peas
½ baked or boiled potato

GRAIN PRODUCTS

KEY VITAMINS: thiamin, riboflavin, niacin, vitamin B_6, and pantothenic acid (necessary to turn food into energy).

One serving is the size of the portion described. Have AT LEAST four servings daily. Limit pastries, doughnuts, and cookies because they are high in fat. Choose whole-grain and enriched products.

- 1 slice whole-grain bread
- ¾ cup ready-to-eat enriched cereal
- ½ cup hot cooked cereal
- 1 pancake or waffle
- ½ cup rice
- ½ cup pasta or noodles
- 2 tortillas
- 1 pita
- 1 muffin or biscuit (higher fat source)
- 4 soda crackers
- 2 rice cakes

FATS AND OILS

KEY VITAMINS: Vitamins A, D, E, K (necessary to protect the body and keep body tissue healthy).

One serving is the size of the portion described. Choose *no more* than four servings daily. Choose unsaturated fats such as oils, mayonnaise, tub margarines, and salad dressings over saturated fats such as butter, lard, stick margarine, or hard shortening because saturated fats raise cholesterol levels and thus the risk of heart disease.

1 tsp any oil
1 tsp margarine
1 tsp mayonnaise
1 Tbsp salad dressing
2 Tbsp nuts or seeds

Keep in mind that although it is smart to get some of each of the five food groups every day, it is not absolutely essential. For at least a short time, your body will store excess quantities of all vitamins for use when vitamin supplies are low. The fat-soluble vitamins are stored almost indefinitely; water-soluble ones are stored for at least a few days. You can pick up the slack for yesterday's poor eating with better food choices today or even correct a whole week of low nutrition in one heavy-duty high-vitamin day of eating. In other words, your vitamin intake can be averaged over a one-week period without causing any health problems. Nevertheless, you will get into trouble if, day after day, week after week, you fail to get all the vitamins you need.

Preserving the Vitamins in Your Food

The following guidelines will help you preserve the vitamins in the food you purchase, store, and prepare.

PURCHASING TO ENHANCE NUTRITIONAL QUALITY

1. Buy whole-grain breads and cereals instead of processed grains to retain the B vitamins. Choose brown rice over white rice.
2. Use milk products that have been fortified with vitamins A and D.
3. Frozen fruits and vegetables may actually retain more vitamins than fresh.
4. Avoid canned fruit and vegetables. The high temperature necessary for canning destroys water-soluble vitamins.
5. Overripe fruits can lose their vitamins.
6. Look for deep rich color and crispness when purchasing fruits or vegetables.
7. Be careful not to choose green potatoes or fruits or vegetables that look spoiled.
8. Frozen meat, poultry, and fish are about as vitamin rich as the fresh varieties.

STORING FOR BETTER VITAMIN RICHNESS

1. Store milk and bread away from the sun or light. Avoid clear glass bottles.
2. Maintain a cool pantry. Do not store canned foods in a hot place.
3. Refrigerate vegetables in moisture-proof containers or crispers. Refrigeration can dry out vegetables.
4. Orange juice will lose vitamin C after several days of storage regardless of the container. Purchase only what you can use in a few days.
5. Allow fruits and vegetables to ripen in a cool dark place.
6. Keep the freezer temperature set at 0 degrees or lower at all times.
7. Do not wash fresh fruit until just before eating.
8. Keep fresh vegetables in their husks, skins, and pods until just before you are ready to use them.

PREPARING THE FRESHEST VITAMINFUL FOODS

1. Don't soak rice or vegetables before cooking. You will lose water-soluble vitamins.
2. Cook vegetables whole rather than in

pieces. Minimize chopping, shredding, and mashing before cooking.

3. Use the shortest cooking time necessary.
4. Cook vegetables until tender. They should be firm, not soft and mushy.
5. Avoid boiling vegetables. Steaming, stir frying, microwaving, or pressure cooking are the best cooking methods. Boiling can remove water-soluble vitamins.
6. If you must boil your vegetables, use a tiny amount of water. Then recycle the water in soups, gravies, or sauces.
7. Cook frozen vegetables frozen. Don't thaw.
8. Rare meat has more thiamin than meats cooked longer. But be careful. If your meat is undercooked, your risk of infectious disease could increase.
9. Broiling meats is better for vitamin retention than stewing or braising.

◆

Vitamin Supplements

VITAMINS: FACT AND FICTION

FICTION: Vitamin pills are a good substitute for a poor diet.

FACT: Vitamin pills contain only a portion of

the many nutrients needed by our bodies or at least the nutrients scientists *know* we need. Many more vitamins may have yet to be discovered. Food also supplies carbohydrates, proteins, and fats as well as fiber and fluids, which are essential for proper digestion and body function. And food is much more fun to eat than a pill!

FICTION: Everyone needs supplemental vitamins to be safe from deficiency.
FACT: For most healthy people who eat a wide variety of nutritious foods from the five food groups, vitamin supplements are unnecessary. The main cause of poor nutrition in the U.S. is misinformation that leads us to make poor food choices from our abundant food supply. Exceptions to this can be found on pages 20–24.

FICTION: Vitamins supply energy to the body.
FACT: Our food energy comes primarily from three sources called macronutrients: carbohydrate, protein, and fat. The fact is that although vitamins enable the macronutrients we eat to work properly, by themselves they have little value.

FICTION: "Natural" vitamins are better than their synthetic counterparts.
FACT: Since vitamins are chemicals, our bodies

can't tell the difference between an expensive, natural chemical and a less expensive laboratory-produced one. No matter what health food stores claim, each vitamin's molecular structure is the same and our bodies use natural and synthetic vitamins identically. Vitamins obtained directly from foods are, of course, the best source since food has many other beneficial ingredients. Incidentally, so-called natural vitamins often contain such synthetic ingredients as dyes, binders, and emulsifiers.

FICTION: Expensive name-brand vitamins are better than store brands.
FACT: The Food and Drug Administration (FDA) regulates the manufacturing and labeling of all vitamins. If a label says each pill contains 100 percent of the RDA for a particular vitamin, whether the bottle cost $1.00 or $10.00 we are getting the same amount of vitamin. We're obviously better off buying the less expensive version and getting our money's worth. By the way, the wholesale cost of a one-month supply of daily vitamins is around 10 cents. Vitamins are big business and mean big profits for manufacturers.

FICTION: If a little bit is good, then a lot must be better.

FACT: Because vitamins are chemicals, there is always a risk when used in large amounts. Too much of a vitamin can be as dangerous as a deficiency. All vitamins should be handled with caution. The RDA for vitamins is based on the amounts the body can use; taking more does no good.

FICTION: Vitamin supplements are best taken in the morning on an empty stomach.
FACT: There is no best time to take a vitamin supplement. Only slight differences in absorption have been found if a supplement is taken with food or on an empty stomach. Take your vitamin supplement when it is most convenient for you, preferably at the same time every day. The only rule is to make sure you store the vitamins in a cool, dry place.

♦

Megadosing: Too Much of a Good Thing?

Megavitamin supplementation is defined as the intake of vitamins at levels at least ten times the RDA. When taken in megadoses, vitamins should be considered drugs rather than food supplements.

WHICH VITAMINS ARE MOST DANGEROUS?

Most nutrition experts agree that vitamin A and D are the most dangerous of all vitamins and shouldn't be taken in large amounts. Like all fat-soluble vitamins, they can accumulate in the body and, in excess quantities, can be toxic. Chronic overdosing of vitamin D can cause calcium deposits in soft body tissue including the heart. Too much vitamin D also can cause growth retardation and kidney damage. Excessive vitamin A can dry out skin and mucous membranes, cause hair loss, and lead to liver damage, growth retardation, and hydrocephalus (water on the brain). A large overdose of either vitamin A or D all at once can kill you. According to some experts, problems can develop at doses as low as five times the RDA. Many widely available vitamin preparations approach that range. The best advice is read the label to make sure that the vitamins do not exceed 100 percent of the RDA. Vitamins E and K, the other fat-soluble vitamins, seem to pose much less of a risk because they are naturally less toxic than vitamins A and D.

Water-soluble vitamins tend to be safer than the fat-soluble ones, but they still can be dangerous at levels that are too high. Although you usually lose an excess of water-soluble vitamins in your urine, your kidneys can process and handle only so much at a time. According to experts, the most dangerous water-soluble vitamins are vitamin B_6 and niacin, although vitamin C and folic acid also can cause problems. Reports indicate that large doses (200 times the RDA) of vitamin B_6 can cause nerve damage, with symptoms ranging from difficulty in walking to numbness in the mouth and hands and the loss of sensory perception.

Although doctors frequently prescribe niacin at levels 100 times the RDA to help lower cholesterol levels, patients must be monitored closely for possible jaundice and liver damage. In addition, large doses of niacin can lead to headaches, cramps, diarrhea, nausea with or without vomiting, flushing of the face and hands (often described as redness with burning and stinging), difficulty metabolizing blood sugar, disturbed heart rhythms, and gouty arthritis. While no one should EVER self-prescribe large doses of any vitamin, this is especially true with vitamin B_6 or niacin.

Vitamin C, once believed to be the safest vitamin, can cause diarrhea, stomachaches, a dry nose, and nosebleeds in doses of 500 mg to 2,000 mg per day. In addition, newborns whose mothers took megadoses of vitamin C during pregnancy will show symptoms of scurvy (a deficiency of vitamin C) after birth. Controversy exists over the research claiming that megadoses of vitamin C can lead to kidney stones and increase the incidence of gout. Think twice before taking large doses of vitamin C this cold and flu season.

In general, folic acid is considered safe in large doses. However, excess folic acid (doses greater than 400 micrograms, or 0.4 mg) can mask pernicious anemia, a severe blood disorder that can cause nerve damage and paralysis if left undiagnosed. In addition, high doses of folic acid may reduce the beneficial action of various anticonvulsant medications in persons with epilepsy.

◆

When Should You Supplement?

Not everyone is able or willing to eat a regular balanced diet. People on weight-loss diets, pregnant and nursing women, strict vegetarians who eat no animal foods at all, and those with stressful, demanding lifestyles (that includes most of us!) may have trouble getting all the vitamins they need in a day.

WEIGHT-LOSS DIETS: WHEN YOU EAT LESS, YOU NEED MORE

If, in an effort to lose weight, you are cutting calories to below 1,200 per day, you will find it difficult to meet all your vitamin needs. No matter how conscious you are about eating healthfully, your intake of vitamins is necessarily cut when you eat such a small amount of food. To ensure proper nutrition, a basic multiple vitamin supplement is recommended. The best over-the-counter vitamin supplements are Centrum, One-a-Day Maximum Formula, and Nature Made Essential Balance. Each is complete and balanced and contains all thirteen vitamins in the proper safe dosage. You may also want to take additional vitamin E, C, and beta carotene for extra protection against heart disease, cancer, and aging in general. Read on for more information about these antioxidant vitamins.

PREGNANT AND NURSING MOTHERS: EATING FOR TWO

During pregnancy, women require more of almost all vitamins but especially of folic acid. Folic acid is required for building new body tissue, including red blood cells. If a woman doesn't get enough folic acid during pregnancy, she may develop a severe blood disorder, megaloblastic anemia. Inadequate folic acid has also been linked to neural tube defects in the baby. In addition, during pregnancy a woman's need for all the B vitamins is increased since her calorie needs are increased. Remember, the B vitamins are involved in regulating energy production from the food we eat. So during pregnancy, when caloric and energy needs are greater, so are B vitamin requirements. Pregnant and nursing women also require extra vitamin D to ensure proper bone and tooth development in the baby.

Although folic aicd and all the other vitamins necessary for a healthy pregnancy can be obtained from a variety of foods, a pregnant woman would need to eat very large amounts to meet her vitamin needs. For this reason, most doctors prescribe a prenatal vitamin supplement to be taken throughout pregnancy and nursing. Research shows that pregnant women who do not take vitamin supplements sometimes experience reduced blood levels of vitamins A, B_6, B_{12}, C, and niacin and are more likely to develop severe vitamin deficiencies. A vitamin-deficient mother may be at greater risk of giving birth to a baby born with a defect.

Helpful Hints for Pregnant Women

1. Never take a prenatal vitamin with more than 5,000 international units (IU) of vitamin A. Too much vitamin A can be toxic to your unborn baby.
2. Avoid taking more vitamin C than is in

your prenatal vitamin. Too much vitamin C can cause the baby to be born with rebound scurvy.

3. If your prenatal vitamin contains iron, take it with a good food source of vitamin C, such as orange or grapefruit juice. Vitamin C enhances the absorption of iron from the intestines into the bloodstream.
4. Never take an iron-containing prenatal vitamin with milk (or other dairy products). Calcium in dairy products prevents proper use of the iron in your supplement.
5. Never take a prenatal vitamin without consulting your doctor first.

STRICT VEGETARIANS: NO ANIMAL PRODUCTS, PLEASE

People who do not eat animal foods may be at risk for vitamin deficiencies. Specifically, vitamins B_{12}, D, and riboflavin may be missing from their diets. Vitamin B_{12} is found *only* in animal foods, and the best sources of vitamin D and riboflavin are dairy products. It is recommended that strict vegetarians supplement these vitamins.

STRESSFUL LIFESTYLES: A SIGN OF THE TIMES

Today many people lead hectic, stressful lives. Eating out, taking home "take out," or preparing convenience foods has become more common than cooking from scratch. Although eating this way can provide lots of calories, if your food choices are not made from a wide variety of foods you will probably not get all the vitamins you need. Careful planning is the key, but who has time to plan? If you eat this way, a multiple vitamin similar to the ones recommended for those on weight-loss diets is recommended.

♦

Choosing the Right Supplement

What to look for:

1. A complete mixture of known vitamins and minerals at or near 100 percent of the RDA. Avoid creating a nutritional imbalance. Never buy a supplement with very large doses of one vitamin or mineral and smaller quantities of others, except as noted below.
2. Beta carotene over vitamin A in supplements. Beta carotene is a safer form of vitamin A found in yellow, orange, and

green fruits and vegetables. Since vitamin A can be toxic in large doses, taking beta carotene makes sense. Beta carotene is also one of the antioxidants. Antioxidants are like rust inhibitors in our bodies and may help prevent some forms of cancer and/or heart disease. For more information on beta carotene, see page 29.

3. Expiration dates. They give some information on potency, although currently there are no regulations guaranteeing that an expiration date has any meaning at all. Most manufacturers, however, typically conduct tests and date supplements to three years beyond manufacture. After this date the vitamin won't harm you but it may have lost some effectiveness.
4. A complete ingredient listing. The more information on the label, the better.
5. Extra vitamin C because vitamin C is one of the antioxidants that may help prevent heart disease, cancer, and cataracts. A supplement with 250 to 500 milligrams of vitamin C is the best. For more information on vitamin C, see pages 27–32.
6. Extra vitamin E because vitamin E is also one of the antioxidants and may not only help prevent heart disease and cancer but also boost the immune system. A supplement with 100 to 400 IU of vitamin E is

best. For more information on vitamin E, see pages 27–32.

7. A supplement with 400 micrograms of folic acid. Most women should get this amount per day. Folic acid may help prevent certain birth defects. Men do not require extra folic acid. For more information on folic acid, see pages 33–34.

What to avoid:

1. Single-nutrient supplementation unless recommended by a physician or registered dietitian. Remember, you want to avoid creating an imbalance of nutrients. High doses of certain nutrients can negate the benefits of others.
2. "Natural" or "organic" supplements. Although these often cost more than synthetic forms, their quality and function are no better. In fact, for example, the body absorbs synthetic folic acid better than the natural form.
3. Amino acids, proteins, and enzymes such as lipase, RNA, beta glutamic acid, taurine, and carnitine. Basically these are added to increase a vitamin's cost. Most diets more than adequately provide all these substances.
4. Unrecognized nutrients such as bioflavi-

noids, biopertin, choline, hydroxyproline, lecithin, myoinositol, orotic acid, PABA, pancreatin, pangamic acid, rutin, and "vitamins" B_{17} and U. These substances, for which no RDA has been established, are not essential in the human diet because some can be made by the body and others have never been found to be necessary to any living being. These substances also add bulk to a supplement, making it hard to swallow.

VITAMIN TAKERS BEWARE: The most frequent cause of poisoning deaths in children is the ingestion of adult iron-containing supplements. Kids also can overdose on children's vitamins. Be sure to keep all supplements out of your child's reach, just as you would with any medication.

♦

What Vitamins Do: Disease Prevention and Health Promotion

BETA CAROTENE AND VITAMINS C AND E: THE ANTIOXIDANT TRIO

What do heart disease, cancer, cataracts, and poor immune function have in common? They all seem to be related to the aging process. As we live longer, our natural immune defenses against disease get weaker and our risk of contracting diseases increases. Current scientific theory suggests that the gradual deterioration of DNA, the body's genetic blueprint, may be responsible for the familiar signs of aging and chronic disease. Now, however, there is reason to believe that some people may age without developing chronic disease conditions. The answer may be in the antioxidants—beta carotene and vitamins C and E—which neutralize free radicals, the molecules that attack the DNA.

Research links vitamin C to an increase in immune function and a decreased risk of cancer, heart disease, and cataracts. Vitamin C also may protect against damage to human sperm. Men with diets deficient in vitamin C seem to have an increased risk of DNA damage in their sperm, thus increasing the risk of birth defects, genetic diseases, and cancer in offspring. Men who smoke should be particularly careful because cigarette smoking decreases blood levels of vitamin C.

Vitamin E also may prevent cataracts and heart disease and reduce the risk of cancer. In addition, vitamin E may decrease the symptoms of the neurologic disorder tardive dyskinesia and specific lung diseases such as bronchitis, asthma, and emphysema. Vitamin E also may boost the immune system.

Beta carotene is associated primarily with an increased immune function and the prevention of cancer and heart disease. Most researchers and physicians are beginning to favor additional supplementation of the antioxidants for this reason. Because optimal levels of each vitamin are still unknown, it may be best, for now, to limit supplementation and get your antioxidants from a healthful diet. High-risk groups such as children, the elderly, and smokers are the prime candidates for any supplementation. Ask your doctor or registered dietitian for more details.

Of course, a nutritious diet low in fat and high in fiber and antioxidants may help reduce disease. Eating more fruits and vegetables rich in antioxidants (at least five servings per day) is always a good idea. Antioxidant supplements shouldn't replace fruits and vegetables, which are naturally low in fat and high in fiber and may contain other as-yet-unidentified nutrients important for disease prevention.

Vitamins alone cannot prevent disease or promote health. For maximum benefit, they need to be used properly in conjunction with an overall healthy eating program and lifestyle.

The following tips are designed to help you live a more healthful life.

To Help Reduce Cancer Risk

1. Reduce total fat in your diet.
2. Eat more high-fiber foods such as fruits, vegetables, whole grains, and legumes.
3. Daily eat at least five servings of fruits and vegetables rich in vitamin C and beta carotene.
4. Choose foods rich in vitamin E.
5. Maintain a desirable body weight.
6. Avoid salt-cured, nitrate-preserved, and smoked foods.
7. Don't smoke.
8. Keep alcohol consumption to a minimum.
9. Avoid excessive sun exposure.

To Help Reduce Heart Disease Risk

1. Reduce total fat and cholesterol in your diet.
2. Eat more foods high in soluble fiber such as legumes, oats, and barley and fruits and vegetables rich in vitamin C and beta carotene.
3. Choose foods rich in vitamin E.
4. Maintain a desirable body weight.

5. Don't smoke.
6. Stay physically active.

To Help Increase Immune Function

1. Reduce total fat in your diet.
2. When you do use fat, choose only olive or canola oil.
3. Daily eat as least five servings of fruits and vegetables rich in vitamin C and beta carotene.
4. Take extra vitamin C when you have a cold. (Be careful not to chew vitamin C tablets: They may erode the enamel on your teeth.)
5. Take a multivitamin daily if you are unable to eat a balanced diet regularly.

Foods Rich in Beta Carotene

apricots
broccoli
cantaloupe
carrots
kale
mangoes
papaya
peaches
pumpkin
spinach
squash (winter and yellow)
sweet potatoes
tomato juice
turnip greens

Foods Rich in Vitamin C

broccoli
brussels sprouts
cantaloupe
cauliflower
collard greens
grapefruit and juice
green pepper
kale
oranges and juice
peppers
potatoes
strawberries
tomatoes and juice
turnip greens

Foods Rich in Vitamin E

green leafy vegetables
liver (high in cholesterol)
nuts (high in fat)
vegetable oils (high in fat)
whole grains
wheat germ

It is difficult to increase vitamin E in the diet without also increasing fat. Try to concentrate on the lowfat, low-cholesterol sources of vitamin E.

VERSATILE VITAMIN B_6

Antioxidants are not the only vitamins capable of decreasing the risk of heart disease and increasing immunity. Vitamin B_6 may also play a role. While most Americans' diets are low in vitamin B_6, because this vitamin can be toxic at even moderate levels (symptoms of overdose include signs of nerve damage), it is recommended that a daily diet include *foods* rich in vitamin B_6 rather than supplements. Such foods include: bananas, brussels sprouts, chicken, fish, lean hamburger, kidney beans, peanuts, lean pork, potatoes, sunflower seeds, walnuts, and whole grains.

Vitamin B_6 has additional benefits for pregnant women. According to a recent study by the University of Iowa College of Medicine, a supplement of 25 milligrams of vitamin B_6 three times per day greatly relieved nausea during pregnancy. If you are pregnant, ask your doctor for more information. NEVER self-prescribe vitamin supplements.

FOLIC ACID AND WOMEN: AN IMPORTANT PAIR

One of the most exciting research discoveries to date on vitamins and disease prevention concerns folic acid (often called folate or folacin) and the prevention of birth defects. Recently, the U.S. Public Health Service recommended that ALL women capable of becoming pregnant supplement their diets with 400 micrograms (0.4 milligrams) of folic acid daily. This would reduce by half the risk of having a baby with a neural tube defect such as spina bifida (incomplete closure of the spinal cord) or anencephaly (no brain). Neural tube defects kill and/or disable nearly 2,500 infants born in the United States each year. Although folic acid is found in a wide variety of foods, a woman would have to eat, for example, more than 1 cup cooked broccoli, 1 medium orange, ¼ melon, ½ cup spinach, AND 2 cups cauliflower every day to satisfy the 400 microgram recommendation. Most women consume foods that contain about half that amount of vitamin B_6.

As with other potentially beneficial vitamins, however, more than the recommended intake is not necessarily better. Excess folic acid can mask such conditions as pernicious anemia, which if left undetected can cause nerve damage and paralysis. To get the recommended 400 micrograms of folic acid each day easily without stuffing yourself, take a regular multivitamin supplement. Most multivitamins contain this amount of the vitamin.

Low blood levels of folic acid also have been linked to an increased risk of cervical cancer and heart disease. So, remember, to reduce your risk of all these diseases, include plenty of folic acid–rich foods in your daily diet. These include: beets, black-eyed peas, brewer's yeast, chicken liver, chick-peas, collard greens, melon, orange juice, orange, and spinach.

VITAMIN D: MAKING STRONG BONES AND PREVENTING COLON CANCER

According to the U.S. Department of Agriculture Human Nutrition Research Center on Aging at Tufts University in Boston, postmenopausal women and older men, especially those living in northern climates, may need a vitamin D supplement during the winter months to prevent bone loss and decrease the risk of osteoporosis (a thinning of the bones). Vitamin D is needed to help absorb calcium from foods. Most vitamin D is obtained from sunlight because human skin can convert sunshine into vitamin D, but in the winter months many people are exposed to less sun. Older skin is also less efficient at making vitamin D than younger skin, and because older people don't get outside as much and are therefore less frequently exposed to the sun, they may require a vitamin D supplement. Senior citizens also are less able to convert vitamin D to a form the body can use and tend to eat less of foods rich in vitamin D.

Fortified milk is one of the best sources of vitamin D. One cup contains 100 IU of vitamin D or half the RDA. Other good sources of vitamin D include: fatty fish such as sardines, salmon, and swordfish and fortified cereals. In addition, getting outdoors ten to fifteen minutes twice a week during the summer months and more often in the winter when the sun is less strong is a good idea. Avoid long exposure to the summer sun, however, because this can increase your risk of skin cancer. If you cannot get out in the sun and the food sources of vitamin D don't appeal to you, ask your doctor if you may take a vitamin D supplement. Four hundred (400) IU a day is considered safe.

Another positive effect of vitamin D may be that it helps protect against colon cancer. Research has shown that people with high blood concentrations of vitamin D have a decreased risk of colon cancer. There also seems to be a higher incidence of colon cancer in parts of the world with the least sunlight.

RIBOFLAVIN (VITAMIN B_2): FOR A NORMAL METABOLISM

A recent study has shown that a woman's need for riboflavin is increased with exercise, since riboflavin helps convert food to energy. For women who exercise regularly, extra riboflavin, above the RDA level, may help maintain normal levels of metabolism. Riboflavin will not, however, increase a slow metabolism or improve exercise performance. To date no studies have been conducted to determine if a man's need for this vitamin also is increased with exercise. To get more riboflavin in your daily diet, eat green leafy vegetables; lowfat milk, cheese, and yogurt; fortified breads and cereals; and lean beef.

VITAMIN B_{12} AND THE ELDERLY

Although most people get more than adequate amounts of vitamin B_{12} in the food they eat (except for strict vegetarians who eat no animal products), a lack of this vitamin may cause many adults over age sixty to exhibit neurologic symptoms ranging from psychiatric disorders, mood changes, disorientation, and memory loss, to weakness, incoordination, and lack of balance. How can this be?

A large percentage of adults over sixty no longer produce enough hydrochloric acid in their stomachs to allow their bodies to use dietary vitamin B_{12}. Without hydrochloric acid, vitamin B_{12} cannot travel from the stomach to the rest of the body where it is needed. To avoid this problem, all that is needed is a simple supplement of vitamin B_{12} (in a pill form) as part of a multivitamin or as a single nutrient, with no more than 100 percent of the RDA. But if you are experiencing problems, *don't* self-prescribe vitamin B_{12} pills. You could lose valuable diagnostic and treatment time if lack of vitamin B_{12} is not the culprit. Furthermore, if the real problem is pernicious anemia due to a lack of intrinsic factor (another substance in the stomach and intestines necessary for the body to absorb and use vitamin B_{12}), no amount of supplementation in pill form will help. People with this problem need to take their B_{12} by injection and avoid the intestinal tract completely.

◆

Sample Menu of a Complete Vitamin Day

Breakfast

1 cup bran flakes cereal
1 cup skim milk
1 fresh peach
4 ounces orange juice

Lunch

2 slices whole-grain bread
½ cup tuna salad made with 1 tsp mayonnaise
romaine lettuce and tomato
1 fresh apple
sparkling water

Snack

4 to 6 whole-wheat crackers
1½ ounces lowfat cheese

Dinner

4 ounces baked skinless chicken
1 cup steamed broccoli
1 medium baked potato with 1 tsp margarine
warm dinner roll
spinach salad with 2 Tbsp Italian dressing
fresh fruit cup
ice water

Snack

1 cup lowfat yogurt (frozen or regular)
1 cup blueberries

♦

Finding the Right Nutrition Counselor

Many people believe that they can create a healthful diet for themselves. But most untrained people just don't know how to choose, prepare, or plan a healthful diet and may end up overly restricting food intake, eliminating entire food groups, or popping vitamin pills instead of eating balanced meals.

Also, although proper nutrition cannot cure illnesses, it can help to manage or prevent certain ones. A nutrition professional will take your health concerns, lifestyle, food preferences, and food allergies into consideration when planning your diet. He or she will be able to help you understand how various foods affect you and determine scientifically whether vitamin supplementation is necessary for you.

If you are searching for a professional, reputable, and responsible nutrition counselor to help you fine-tune your vitamin and nutrition intake, your best bet is to consult a registered dietitian (R.D.). The R.D. designation guarantees that the practitioner has obtained at least a bachelor's degree in nutrition from an accredited college or university, completed an internship in a hospital or clinic, and passed a national certification exam. R.D.s also must keep their knowledge current with yearly continuing education. Many R.D.s have master's degrees or Ph.D.s and often have specialty training in various medical areas, such as diabetes, eating disorders, and maternal and child nutrition.

Keep in mind that anyone can call him- or herself a nutritionist. The R.D. signals professional training. An R.D. may call him- or herself a nutritionist, but it is illegal for a nutritionist to call him- or herself an R.D. Some states also have licensure laws that can help you find a qualified nutrition counselor. Look for the terms licensed dietitian (L.D.) or licensed nutritionist (L.N.) if your state requires licensing of nutrition professionals.

To find an R.D. or licensed professional, first try the yellow pages under nutritionist or dietitians. Another good resource is the American Dietetic Association in Chicago at 1-800-877-1600. A dietitian can evaluate your personal eating habits and patterns, make recommendations, and guide you to better health. If you need specific tests run, such as blood work or a urinalysis, or if you have a nutrition-related disease such as diabetes or heart disease, try to find an R.D. associated with your doctor. A complete nutrition evaluation will cost $60 to $200 depending on where you live.

Avoid any "nutritionist" who sells vitamins or other dietary supplements, offers hair analysis or applied kinesiology and iridology to evaluate nutrition status, recommends similar regimens for all clients, claims that without supplements it is impossible to get a balanced diet, pushes a quick fix for weight loss and other complaints, eliminates entire food groups, or recommends fasting to rid the body of toxins.

VITAMINS AT A GLANCE

Vitamins	Deficiency Signs	Known and Potential Health Benefits	Best Dietary Sources
Vitamin A	Night blindness, diarrhea, intestinal infections, impaired growth	Increases resistance to infections, promotes bone and tooth development	Butter, cheese, eggs, liver, milk
Beta carotene	None documented	May lower risk of heart disease and cancer, slow the development of cataracts, and boost the immune system	Dark-green leafy vegetables, yellow and orange fruits and vegetables

Vitamin B_1 (Thiamin)	Impaired growth, mental confusion, depression (beriberi)	Promotes normal metabolism, appetite, and nervous system function	Fortified grains, legumes, liver, meats, nuts, pork, whole grains
Vitamin B_2 (Riboflavin)	Cracks at the corner of the mouth, eye problems	Promotes energy release from food, good vision, and healthy skin. May help maintain normal metabolism in women who exercise	Beef, cheese, fortified grains, green leafy vegetables, milk, yogurt

Vitamins	Deficiency Signs	Known and Potential Health Benefits	Best Dietary Sources
Vitamin B_3 (Niacin)	Weakness, skin and intestinal problems, loss of appetite, irritability, dizziness (pellagra)	Promotes normal metabolism; healthy skin, nerves, and intestines; normal appetite and digestion. In large doses, when prescribed by a physician, helps lower cholesterol	Fish, fortified grains, meat, peanuts, poultry
Vitamin B_6	Neurological abnormalities, anemia, skin problems	Assists in the formation of red blood cells and in normal fat and protein metabolism. May decrease risk of heart	Bananas, chicken, eggs, fish, liver, oats, peanuts, pork, potatoes, soybeans, walnuts, whole wheat

		disease and increase immune function. May help reduce nausea in pregnancy	
Vitamin B_{12}	Pernicious anemia, neurological disorders	Promotes normal red blood cell metabolism, and maintenance of nerves. May help reduce neurologic symptoms in the elderly	Dairy products, eggs, fish, meat, poultry

Vitamins	Deficiency Signs	Known and Potential Health Benefits	Best Dietary Sources
Vitamin C	Easy bruising, bleeding gums, scruvy	Strengthens blood vessels, increases wound healing and resistance to infections. May reduce risk of cancer, heart disease, and cataracts. May boost the immune system and protect against damage to human sperm	Broccoli, brussels sprouts, collard greens, grapefruit, oranges and juice, papaya, strawberries, sweet and hot peppers, tangerines, tomatoes
Vitamin D	Soft bones and teeth (rickets and osteomalacia)	Increases intestinal absorption of calcium, builds strong bones and teeth. May help	Eggs, fish, fortified milk, liver. Sunlight is the best source.

		prevent osteoporosis in the elderly and protect against colon cancer	
Vitamin E	(RARE) Reproductive failure, anemia in low-birthweight infants	Prevents cell damage. May lower risk of heart disease and cancer. May help the body fight infections and protect against cataracts. May decrease symptoms of certain neurological and lung diseases	Dark-green leafy vegetables, eggs, nuts, wheat germ, whole-grain cereals, vegetable oils

Vitamins	Deficiency Signs	Known and Potential Health Benefits	Best Dietary Sources
Vitamin K	(RARE) Excessive bleeding	Helps to clot the blood and may help prevent osteoporosis	Cereals, dairy products, eggs, fruits, green leafy vegetables, meats, vegetables. Also produced in the intestines.
Biotin	Fatigue, depression, nausea, skin problems, muscle pain	Promotes normal metabolism	Eggs, milk, organ meats, most fresh vegetables

Folic Acid	Diarrhea, anemia, irritability, red tongue	Promotes red blood cell formation and protein metabolism. May help reduce risk of birth defects, cervical cancer, and heart disease	Beets, black-eyed peas, brewer's yeast, chicken livers, chick-peas, collard greens, orange juice, spinach
Pantothenic Acid	(RARE) Fatigue, sleep disturbances, nausea	Promotes normal metabolism	Eggs, legumes, milk, organ meats, whole grains